UNLOCKING HEMOCHROMATOSIS

A Comprehensive Guide to
Managing Iron Overload Through
Diet and Lifestyle

Adams .U. Morris

TABLE OF CONTENTS

CHAPTER 1

Introduction
Hemochromatosis

Hemochromatosis, often referred to as "iron overload," is a condition that affects how the body absorbs and stores iron. This chapter aims to provide a comprehensive understanding of hemochromatosis, including its causes, effects on the body, and why diet plays a crucial role in managing it.

The Basics of Hemochromatosis

Imagine iron as an essential mineral in your body, which it is. Iron helps carry oxygen through your bloodstream, enabling your cells and organs to function properly. But, like many things in life, too much of a good thing can be harmful. This is where hemochromatosis comes into play.

Hemochromatosis is a genetic disorder that affects the way your body absorbs and regulates iron. Normally, your body absorbs just enough iron from the food you eat to meet its needs. However, individuals with hemochromatosis have a genetic mutation that causes their bodies to absorb excessive amounts of iron from their diet. This iron buildup can be problematic because your body has no efficient way to get rid of excess iron. As a result, the excess iron accumulates in your organs, particularly the liver, heart, and pancreas, and can lead to a host of health problems.

Genetic and Environmental Factors

Hemochromatosis is primarily a genetic condition. It is most common in people of Northern European descent, particularly those of Celtic origin. The genetic mutations associated with hemochromatosis are more prevalent in these populations. However, it's essential to note that not everyone with these genetic mutations will develop hemochromatosis. The condition often requires specific combinations of these mutations to manifest.

Genetics isn't the whole story, though. Environmental factors can influence how hemochromatosis manifests. For example, dietary choices can exacerbate or mitigate the effects of the condition. Certain lifestyle factors, such as alcohol consumption and other health conditions, can also play a role in the progression of hemochromatosis.

The Impact of Excess Iron

So, what's the big deal about having too much iron in your body? Excess iron can wreak havoc on your organs and overall health. Here's how:

1. **Liver Damage**: The liver is responsible for regulating iron levels in the body. When excess iron accumulates in the liver, it can lead to liver damage,

cirrhosis, and even liver cancer.

2. **Heart Problems**: Iron buildup in the heart can lead to a condition called cardiomyopathy, where the heart muscle becomes weak and less effective at pumping blood.

3. **Diabetes**: Hemochromatosis can increase the risk of developing type 2 diabetes, as excess iron can damage the pancreas, which produces insulin.

4. **Joint Pain**: Some people with hemochromatosis

experience joint pain, often misdiagnosed as arthritis, due to iron deposits in the joints.

5. **Skin Changes**: Iron buildup can cause changes in skin color, leading to a bronze or grayish tint.

6. **Fatigue and Weakness**: Excess iron can interfere with normal bodily functions, leading to fatigue, weakness, and a general feeling of unwellness.

The Role of Diet

Now that we understand the basics of hemochromatosis, let's delve into why diet is a crucial aspect of managing this condition. While hemochromatosis is genetic, dietary choices can significantly influence the severity and progression of the condition. What you eat directly affects the amount of iron your body absorbs, so it's an essential factor to consider in your management plan.

In simple terms, individuals with hemochromatosis need to be mindful of their iron intake because their bodies tend to absorb more iron than they need. This means they should avoid excessive consumption of iron-rich foods and make specific dietary adjustments to prevent further iron buildup.

This chapter sets the stage for the rest of the book by establishing the importance of understanding hemochromatosis and its relationship with diet. It lays the foundation for readers to grasp the significance of dietary choices in managing this condition effectively.

CHAPTER 2

Diagnosis and Treatment Options

How Hemochromatosis is Diagnosed

Diagnosing hemochromatosis can be a complex process but is crucial for effective management. The journey usually begins with recognizing symptoms or screening due to a family history of the condition. Common symptoms of hemochromatosis include fatigue, joint pain, abdominal pain, and changes in skin color, among others.

If you or your healthcare provider suspect hemochromatosis, several diagnostic tests can confirm or rule out the condition:

1. **Blood Tests**: Blood tests are the first step in diagnosing hemochromatosis. They measure your serum ferritin levels (a protein that stores iron) and transferrin saturation (a measure of how much iron your body is using). Elevated levels of

these markers can indicate hemochromatosis.

2. **Genetic Testing**: Genetic testing can identify specific mutations associated with hemochromatosis, providing a definitive diagnosis. This is particularly useful for individuals with a family history of the condition.

3. **Liver Biopsy**: In some cases, a liver biopsy may be performed to assess the extent of iron buildup in the liver and to check for liver damage.

Stages and Severity of the Condition

Hemochromatosis is not a one-size-fits-all condition. Its severity can vary from person to person. To better understand the condition's progression and how to manage it, it's important to be aware of its stages:

1. **Asymptomatic Stage**: In the early stages, individuals with hemochromatosis may not experience noticeable symptoms. However, excess iron is still accumulating in their organs.

2. **Symptomatic Stage**: As iron levels continue to rise, symptoms may begin to manifest. These can include fatigue, joint pain, abdominal pain, and skin changes.

3. **Organ Damage Stage**: If left untreated, hemochromatosis can lead to organ damage, particularly in the liver, heart, and pancreas. This is why early diagnosis and intervention are crucial.

Medical Treatments and Phlebotomy

Once hemochromatosis is diagnosed, medical intervention becomes essential to manage iron levels and prevent further damage. One of the most common treatments for hemochromatosis is phlebotomy, also known as therapeutic bloodletting.

Phlebotomy is a straightforward procedure that involves removing a specific amount of blood, usually around 500 milliliters, at regular intervals. This process effectively reduces the iron load in the body because iron is stored in red blood cells. Over time, this helps bring iron levels back to normal.

The frequency of phlebotomy sessions varies from person to person and depends on the severity of the condition. Initially, sessions may be frequent, such as once a week, but they can become less frequent as iron levels normalize.

The Role of Diet Alongside Medical Interventions

While medical treatments like phlebotomy are crucial for managing hemochromatosis, they are most effective when combined with dietary adjustments. This is where the concept of a hemochromatosis-friendly diet comes into play, which will be explored in greater detail in subsequent chapters.

The reason diet is so important in the management of hemochromatosis is that it can help reduce the need for frequent phlebotomies. By

CHAPTER 3

Iron-Rich Foods to Avoid

In this chapter, we will delve into the foods that individuals with hemochromatosis should avoid or consume in moderation due to their high iron content. Understanding these foods is essential for managing the condition effectively, as it helps reduce the risk of further iron accumulation in the body.

Iron Absorption and Types of Dietary Iron

Before we dive into the specific foods to avoid, it's crucial to understand the two main types of dietary iron: heme and non-heme iron. This distinction is essential because the body absorbs these two forms of iron differently.

Heme Iron: This type of iron is found in animal-based foods, primarily in red meat, such as beef, lamb, and pork. Heme iron is absorbed more efficiently by the body compared to non-heme iron. This means that even small servings of heme iron-rich foods can significantly contribute to iron intake.

Non-Heme Iron: Non-heme iron is found in plant-based foods and fortified foods. While the body doesn't absorb non-heme iron as effectively as heme iron, it still contributes to overall iron intake. Some common sources of non-heme iron include beans, lentils, tofu, fortified cereals, and spinach.

Foods to Avoid or Limit

1. **Red Meat**: As mentioned earlier, red meat is a significant source of heme iron. For individuals with hemochromatosis, it's essential to limit

consumption of beef, lamb, pork, and other red meats.

2. **Organ Meats**: Organ meats, such as liver, kidney, and heart, are exceptionally high in iron and should be strictly avoided by individuals with hemochromatosis.

3. **Shellfish**: Shellfish like clams, mussels, and oysters are rich in heme iron and should be consumed sparingly.

4. **Iron-Fortified Foods**: While fortified foods can be a valuable source of nutrients for some people,

they can contribute to excess iron intake in individuals with hemochromatosis. Check food labels for iron fortification, especially in breakfast cereals and plant-based meat substitutes.

5. **Supplements with Iron**: Some dietary supplements contain iron. It's crucial for individuals with hemochromatosis to avoid iron supplements unless specifically recommended by a healthcare provider.

6. **Cookware**: The type of cookware used can also influence iron intake. Cast

iron cookware, for instance, can leach iron into the food being cooked. It's advisable to use alternative cookware materials like stainless steel or non-stick pans.

7. **Alcohol**: While not a food, alcohol can increase the absorption of dietary iron. It's advisable for individuals with hemochromatosis to limit alcohol consumption or, ideally, abstain from alcohol altogether.

Understanding Iron Content in Foods

To effectively manage iron intake, individuals with hemochromatosis should be diligent about reading food labels and familiarizing themselves with the iron content of common foods. Food labels often provide information about the percentage of the recommended daily intake (RDI) of iron per serving. Keep in mind that the RDI for iron is based on the needs of the general population, not individuals with hemochromatosis, who should aim for much lower iron intake.

It's also essential to recognize that portion sizes matter. Even foods with moderate iron content can contribute significantly to iron intake if consumed in large quantities.

Practical Tips for Reducing Iron Intake

Managing iron intake can be challenging, but it's crucial for individuals with hemochromatosis. Here are some practical tips to help reduce iron intake:

1. **Portion Control**: Be mindful of portion sizes, especially when consuming foods high in heme iron.

Smaller servings can help reduce iron intake.

2. **Food Preparation**: Trim visible fat from meat before cooking, as iron tends to accumulate in fatty tissues. Additionally, cooking meat until it's well-done can decrease its iron content.

3. **Dietary Diversity**: Incorporate a variety of foods into your diet to ensure balanced nutrition while reducing reliance on iron-rich sources.

4. **Vegetarian and Vegan Options**: If you're open to plant-based diets, explore

vegetarian and vegan sources of protein like beans, lentils, tofu, and tempeh. These foods provide non-heme iron, which is absorbed less efficiently than heme iron.

5. **Iron-Free Snacking**: Choose low-iron snacks like fresh fruits, vegetables, and nuts when you need a quick bite.

6. **Limit Caffeine with Meals**: Caffeine can slightly inhibit iron absorption, so consider limiting caffeinated beverages during meals.

7. **Cooking Methods**: Use cooking methods that minimize iron absorption, such as boiling, stewing, and steaming, rather than frying.

CHAPTER 4

Creating a Hemochromatosis-Friendly Diet

Now that we've covered the foods to avoid, let's focus on creating a diet that's tailored to individuals with hemochromatosis. This diet aims to strike a balance between meeting nutritional needs and minimizing iron intake.

Designing a Balanced and Nutritious Diet

It's essential to emphasize that managing hemochromatosis through diet doesn't mean sacrificing overall nutrition. With careful planning, individuals with hemochromatosis can enjoy a balanced and nutritious diet. Here are some key components to consider when designing a hemochromatosis-friendly diet:

1. **Protein Sources**: Since red meat and organ meats are restricted, explore alternative protein sources like poultry (chicken and turkey), fish (preferably non-oily varieties), eggs, dairy

products, and plant-based options like legumes (beans, lentils, chickpeas), tofu, and tempeh.

2. **Fruits and Vegetables**: Incorporate a wide variety of fruits and vegetables into your diet. These foods are rich in essential vitamins and minerals and can provide antioxidants that support overall health.

3. **Whole Grains**: Choose whole grains like brown rice, quinoa, whole wheat pasta, and oats to provide fiber and energy.

4. **Dairy or Dairy Alternatives**: Dairy products can be an excellent source of calcium and protein. If you're lactose intolerant or prefer non-dairy options, choose fortified plant-based milks (such as almond, soy, or oat milk) and yogurts.

5. **Healthy Fats**: Include sources of healthy fats in your diet, such as avocados, nuts, seeds, and olive oil.

6. **Iron-Free Snacks**: Keep iron-free snacks like fresh fruits, vegetables, and

unsalted nuts on hand for healthy munching.

7. **Hydration**: Drink plenty of water throughout the day to stay hydrated. Adequate hydration supports overall health and can aid in digestion.

Portion Control and Meal Planning

Portion control is a crucial aspect of managing hemochromatosis through diet. Smaller portions of iron-rich foods help keep iron intake in check. Consider the following portion control strategies:

1. **Use Smaller Plates**: Opt for smaller plates and bowls to help control portion sizes naturally.

2. **Plan Balanced Meals**: Plan your meals to include a variety of foods from different food groups. This helps ensure you get a range of nutrients without relying heavily on a single iron-rich source.

3. **Measure Ingredients**: When cooking, use measuring cups and spoons to portion out ingredients accurately.

4. **Eat Mindfully**: Pay attention to your body's hunger and fullness cues. Eating slowly and savoring each bite can help prevent overeating.

Recipes and Meal Ideas

To make meal planning easier for individuals with hemochromatosis, this chapter can include a selection of recipes and meal ideas that adhere to the dietary guidelines outlined in the previous sections. These recipes can be diverse and appealing, catering to different tastes and dietary preferences.

Sample recipes could include:

1. **Grilled Lemon Herb Chicken with Quinoa Salad**: A lean protein source with a quinoa salad loaded with vegetables.

2. **Vegetarian Chili**: A hearty chili made with beans, vegetables, and spices for flavor.

3. **Baked Salmon with Roasted Vegetables**: A nutritious meal rich in omega-3 fatty acids and antioxidants.

4. **Spinach and Chickpea Salad**: A light and

nutritious salad with spinach, chickpeas, and a citrus vinaigrette.

5. **Tofu Stir-Fry**: A flavorful stir-fry with tofu, a variety of colorful vegetables, and a ginger-soy sauce.

These recipes should be adaptable to individual preferences and dietary restrictions, such as vegetarian or gluten-free diets.

Additional Considerations

It's important to highlight that dietary needs can vary from person to person, and individualized guidance from a healthcare provider or registered dietitian can be immensely valuable. A dietitian with experience in hemochromatosis can help create a personalized nutrition plan that considers specific iron levels, health goals, and dietary preferences.

This chapter should also address the importance of regular monitoring of iron levels through blood tests to ensure that dietary adjustments are effectively managing the condition. It can emphasize that dietary changes, in conjunction with other medical treatments, play a vital role in maintaining optimal health and preventing complications related to hemochromatosis.

By the end of this chapter, readers should have a clear understanding of how to structure their diets to manage hemochromatosis effectively, including practical meal ideas and portion control strategies.

CHAPTER 5

Nutritional Supplements and Medications

In this chapter, we will explore the role of nutritional supplements and medications in managing hemochromatosis. While dietary adjustments are a crucial aspect of managing this condition, they may not be sufficient on their own. Supplements and medications can complement dietary changes and help regulate iron levels effectively.

The Use of Supplements

Supplements can be beneficial for individuals with hemochromatosis, but they should be used judiciously and under the guidance of a healthcare provider. Here are some supplements commonly considered in the management of hemochromatosis:

1. **Vitamin C**: Vitamin C can enhance the absorption of non-heme iron, the type of iron found in plant-based foods and fortified products. While this might seem counterintuitive for individuals with hemochromatosis, who are

trying to reduce iron absorption, vitamin C can be strategically used to increase iron absorption when necessary. However, it's crucial to use vitamin C supplements with caution and only under the guidance of a healthcare provider.

2. **Calcium**: Calcium can inhibit the absorption of dietary iron. Including calcium-rich foods in your diet or taking calcium supplements with meals can help reduce iron absorption. Again, it's essential to consult a healthcare

provider before adding calcium supplements to your regimen.

3. **Tannins**: Tannins are compounds found in tea, coffee, and red wine. They can also inhibit iron absorption when consumed with iron-rich foods. While these beverages should generally be consumed in moderation due to other potential health concerns, they can be strategically included in the diet to help reduce iron absorption when necessary.

4. **Phytic Acid**: Phytic acid is found in foods like whole grains, legumes, and nuts. It can also inhibit iron absorption. Including these foods in your diet can help manage iron levels effectively.

It's important to reiterate that the use of supplements should be personalized and based on your specific iron levels and overall health. Self-prescribing supplements without professional guidance can lead to unintended consequences, including nutrient imbalances.

Medications to Aid in Iron Absorption Regulation

In some cases, healthcare providers may recommend medications to further assist in regulating iron absorption. These medications can be particularly useful when dietary adjustments and phlebotomy alone are insufficient in managing iron levels. Here are some medications commonly used:

1. **Iron Chelators**: Iron chelators are medications that bind to excess iron in the body, effectively removing it. Common iron

chelators include deferoxamine, deferiprone, and deferasirox. These medications are typically reserved for individuals with severe iron overload or those who cannot undergo phlebotomy.

2. **Anti-Inflammatory Medications**:

Inflammatory conditions can increase iron absorption. Therefore, individuals with hemochromatosis who also have inflammatory conditions may benefit from medications that reduce inflammation, such as nonsteroidal anti-inflammatory drugs (NSAIDs).

3. **Hepatitis C Treatment**: For individuals with hemochromatosis who also have hepatitis C, successful treatment of hepatitis C can lead to improved liver health and potentially reduce iron overload.

Dosages, Risks, and Benefits

The dosages and duration of supplements and medications should be determined by a healthcare provider based on your specific needs and response to treatment. It's essential to follow their guidance closely and have regular follow-up appointments to monitor the effectiveness of these interventions.

While supplements and medications can be valuable tools in managing hemochromatosis, they are not without risks. Potential risks and considerations include:

1. **Side Effects**: Some medications used to manage hemochromatosis, particularly iron chelators, can have side effects. These may include gastrointestinal

symptoms, joint pain, or skin rashes.

2. **Interactions**: Supplements and medications can interact with other drugs you may be taking. It's crucial to inform your healthcare provider of all the medications and supplements you are using to avoid potentially harmful interactions.

3. **Monitoring**: Regular monitoring of iron levels, liver function, and overall health is essential when using supplements and medications. This ensures

that treatment is effective and safe.

4. **Individual Response**: Everyone's response to supplements and medications can vary. What works for one person may not be as effective for another. It's important to communicate openly with your healthcare provider about how you are feeling and any changes in your health.

5. **Cost**: Some of the medications used to manage hemochromatosis can be expensive. Be sure to discuss

the cost and potential insurance coverage with your healthcare provider.

In summary, supplements and medications can be valuable additions to the management of hemochromatosis, but their use should be individualized, carefully monitored, and guided by healthcare professionals who are familiar with the condition.

CHAPTER 6

Lifestyle Changes and Management

Managing hemochromatosis effectively involves more than dietary adjustments and medical treatments. Lifestyle changes play a significant role in controlling iron levels and maintaining overall health. This chapter explores various lifestyle factors that can impact hemochromatosis and offers guidance on how to make positive changes.

Alcohol Consumption and Hemochromatosis

Alcohol consumption is a crucial lifestyle factor to consider when managing hemochromatosis. Alcohol can have several effects on iron metabolism:

1. **Increased Iron Absorption**: Alcohol consumption has been associated with increased absorption of dietary iron, which can exacerbate iron overload in individuals with hemochromatosis.

2. **Liver Health**: Excessive alcohol intake can harm the

liver, leading to conditions like alcoholic liver disease. When combined with hemochromatosis, which also affects the liver, the risk of liver damage becomes more significant.

Given these concerns, it's advisable for individuals with hemochromatosis to limit or, ideally, abstain from alcohol altogether. If you find it challenging to reduce or eliminate alcohol from your life, consider seeking support from healthcare providers or support groups to help you make this important lifestyle change.

The Role of Regular Exercise

Regular physical activity is an essential component of a healthy lifestyle for individuals with hemochromatosis. Exercise offers several benefits:

1. **Liver Health**: Exercise can support liver health by reducing fat accumulation and inflammation in the liver.

2. **Improved Insulin Sensitivity**: Hemochromatosis is

associated with an increased risk of developing type 2 diabetes. Exercise can improve insulin sensitivity and help manage blood sugar levels.

3. **Weight Management**: Maintaining a healthy weight is important for managing hemochromatosis, as excess body fat can contribute to inflammation and insulin resistance.

4. **Cardiovascular Health**: Regular exercise can improve cardiovascular health, which is especially important for individuals

with hemochromatosis, as they may be at a higher risk of heart problems due to iron overload.

When incorporating exercise into your routine, aim for a combination of cardiovascular activities (such as walking, jogging, or cycling) and strength training exercises. However, it's essential to start slowly and consult with your healthcare provider, especially if you have any underlying health conditions or concerns.

Stress Management and Its Impact on Iron Levels

Stress is a common part of modern life, but excessive or chronic stress can have negative effects on overall health, including iron metabolism. Stress hormones can affect the body's ability to regulate iron absorption and utilization. Therefore, effective stress management is crucial for individuals with hemochromatosis.

Here are some stress management strategies to consider:

1. **Mindfulness and Relaxation Techniques**: Practices like meditation, deep breathing, and

progressive muscle relaxation can help reduce stress levels.

2. **Regular Physical Activity**: Exercise is not only beneficial for physical health but also for managing stress and promoting mental well-being.

3. **Counseling or Therapy**: Talking to a mental health professional can be helpful in developing coping strategies and managing stress.

4. **Time Management**: Organizing your time and priorities can help reduce

stress related to work, family, and other responsibilities.

5. **Social Support**: Maintaining strong social connections and seeking support from friends and family can be invaluable in times of stress.

Monitoring and Tracking Your Progress

To effectively manage hemochromatosis and the lifestyle changes associated with it, monitoring and tracking your progress are essential. This can include:

1. **Regular Medical Checkups**: Schedule regular checkups with your healthcare provider to monitor iron levels, liver function, and overall health. These appointments provide an opportunity to discuss any concerns or adjustments to your treatment plan.

2. **Keeping a Health Journal**: Consider keeping a journal to track your diet, exercise routines, and stress levels. This can help you identify patterns and make informed decisions about your lifestyle.

3. **Self-Care Routine**: Develop a self-care routine that includes healthy eating, regular exercise, stress management, and adequate sleep. Consistency in these areas can lead to better overall health.

4. **Support Groups**: Consider joining a support group for individuals with hemochromatosis. These groups can provide a sense of community, shared experiences, and valuable information.

Conclusion of Chapter 6

In this chapter, we've explored how lifestyle changes can significantly impact the management of hemochromatosis. By making informed choices regarding alcohol consumption, incorporating regular exercise, and managing stress effectively, individuals with hemochromatosis can complement their medical treatments and dietary adjustments, ultimately improving their quality of life and reducing the risk of complications associated with iron overload.

This chapter serves as a reminder that hemochromatosis

management is a holistic approach that encompasses various aspects of life. It's not just about what you eat or the medications you take; it's also about how you live and care for your overall well-being. Effective management requires a combination of medical guidance, dietary adjustments, and lifestyle changes to maintain optimal health and prevent the progression of this condition.

CHAPTER 7

Cooking and Food Preparation Tips

In this chapter, we'll dive into cooking and food preparation strategies tailored to individuals with hemochromatosis. These tips are designed to help you create delicious, satisfying meals while keeping your iron intake in check.

Cooking Methods that Reduce Iron Absorption

1. **Boiling**: Boiling is an effective cooking method for

reducing iron content in foods. When you boil food, some of the iron leaches into the cooking water, reducing the iron content of the food itself. For example, when cooking vegetables, consider blanching them in boiling water for a short time before consuming.

2. **Steaming**: Steaming is another excellent way to retain nutrients while reducing iron content. Vegetables, in particular, benefit from steaming, as this method preserves their

color and texture while minimizing iron absorption.

3. **Stewing**: Stewing involves simmering food in liquid over a longer period. This can be a great way to prepare lean cuts of meat or poultry, as the extended cooking time allows some of the iron to leach into the liquid.

4. **Crockpot Cooking**: Slow cookers or crockpots are excellent for preparing meals with minimal effort. When using a crockpot, consider recipes that include vegetables, legumes, and lean meats. The prolonged

cooking process can help reduce iron content.

Choosing Cookware Wisely

The type of cookware you use can influence the iron content of your meals. Here's what you need to know:

1. **Cast Iron Cookware**: While cast iron cookware is renowned for its excellent heat retention and even cooking, it can also transfer iron to the food being prepared. If you prefer using cast iron, reserve it for dishes that are low in iron

content or use alternative cookware for iron-sensitive meals.

2. **Stainless Steel Cookware**: Stainless steel pots and pans are a suitable choice for individuals with hemochromatosis. They do not transfer iron to the food, ensuring that your meals remain lower in iron content.

3. **Non-Stick Cookware**: Non-stick cookware with a Teflon or ceramic coating is also a good option. These surfaces prevent food from

sticking and don't introduce iron into your dishes.

4. **Glass and Ceramic Bakeware**: When baking, consider using glass or ceramic bakeware. These materials do not contain iron and are ideal for recipes like casseroles or baked dishes.

Food Storage and Handling Practices

Proper food storage and handling can help maintain the nutritional quality of your meals while minimizing iron exposure:

1. **Refrigeration**: Store leftover foods in the refrigerator promptly. Cold storage can slow down the oxidation process, which can lead to increased iron absorption from stored foods.

2. **Avoid Cooking in Iron Pots**: If you have cast iron cookware, avoid cooking acidic foods like tomato-based sauces, as they can increase the amount of iron transferred to the food.

3. **Use Airtight Containers**: When storing prepared meals or ingredients, use

airtight containers to prevent exposure to oxygen, which can accelerate iron oxidation.

4. **Prevent Cross-Contamination**: When handling raw meat, poultry, or fish, use separate cutting boards and utensils to prevent cross-contamination. This practice reduces the risk of unintentional iron exposure from these sources.

5. **Cook Fresh Whenever Possible**: While leftovers can be convenient, cooking fresh meals can help you

have more control over the ingredients and their iron content.

Adapting Recipes for Lower Iron Intake

You don't need to give up your favorite recipes entirely. Instead, adapt them to reduce their iron content:

1. **Use Lean Cuts of Meat**: When a recipe calls for meat, opt for lean cuts like chicken breast, turkey, or lean beef. These cuts generally have less iron than fattier options.

2. **Trim Fat**: If you do use meat, trim any visible fat before cooking. Iron accumulates in fatty tissues, so removing excess fat can help reduce iron content.

3. **Add Iron-Reducing Ingredients**: Incorporate ingredients known to inhibit iron absorption into your recipes. For instance, consider adding foods high in calcium, like low-fat cheese or yogurt, or sources of tannins, such as tea or coffee, depending on the dish.

4. **Limit Iron-Rich Ingredients**: Be mindful of ingredients that are naturally high in iron, like spinach or certain legumes. Use them in moderation or explore alternatives when possible.

5. **Explore Meat Alternatives**: Try plant-based meat alternatives like tofu, tempeh, or seitan in recipes that traditionally call for meat.

6. **Experiment with International Cuisine**: Explore cuisines from regions with naturally lower-

iron diets, such as Asian or Mediterranean dishes. These cuisines often feature ingredients and cooking methods that can align with your dietary needs.

By implementing these cooking and food preparation tips, you can continue to enjoy a wide range of delicious meals while managing your hemochromatosis effectively.

CHAPTER 8

Living Well with Hemochromatosis

In the final chapter of this book, we will focus on the holistic aspects of living well with hemochromatosis. This includes personal stories, coping strategies, support systems, and looking ahead to the future of managing this condition.

Success Stories and Testimonials

Personal stories and testimonials from individuals who have

successfully managed hemochromatosis can provide inspiration and hope to those newly diagnosed or currently navigating the condition. These stories can offer insights into the challenges and triumphs associated with living with hemochromatosis.

Success stories might include individuals who have effectively managed their iron levels through dietary adjustments, phlebotomy, and lifestyle changes. They can also highlight the importance of regular medical monitoring and the support they've received from healthcare providers, friends, and family.

Coping with the Emotional Impact

Living with a chronic condition like hemochromatosis can take a toll on one's emotional well-being. It's essential to address the emotional impact and provide strategies for coping with the challenges it presents:

1. **Educate Yourself**: Understanding your condition and its management is empowering. Knowledge reduces anxiety

and helps you make informed decisions.

2. **Seek Support**: Don't hesitate to reach out to support groups or connect with others who have hemochromatosis. Sharing experiences and advice can be invaluable.

3. **Talk to a Therapist**: A mental health professional can help you navigate the emotional aspects of living with hemochromatosis, from anxiety and depression to stress management.

4. **Lean on Your Support System**: Friends and family

can be a significant source of emotional support. Open communication and sharing your experiences with loved ones can strengthen your emotional well-being.

5. **Set Realistic Goals**: Setting achievable goals, both in managing your condition and in your personal life, can boost your confidence and sense of control.

6. **Practice Mindfulness**: Mindfulness techniques, such as meditation and deep breathing exercises, can help

reduce stress and promote emotional resilience.

Support Groups and Resources

Support groups and resources play a vital role in helping individuals with hemochromatosis navigate their journey. These resources can provide information, guidance, and a sense of community:

1. **Local Support Groups**: Many regions have local support groups for individuals with hemochromatosis. These groups offer a space to share experiences, ask questions,

and find local healthcare providers familiar with the condition.

2. **Online Communities**: Online forums and social media groups can connect you with people worldwide who are dealing with hemochromatosis. These communities provide a platform for discussion, information sharing, and emotional support.

3. **Educational Materials**: Books, websites, and organizations dedicated to hemochromatosis can provide valuable information

about the condition, treatment options, and lifestyle management.

4. **Patient Advocacy Groups**: Consider getting involved with patient advocacy groups focused on hemochromatosis. These organizations often work to raise awareness, promote research, and provide support to those affected by the condition.

Looking Ahead: Advances in Hemochromatosis Management

The final section of this chapter can touch on the future of hemochromatosis management. Medical research is continually advancing, and there may be promising developments on the horizon. Highlighting these advances can instill hope and optimism for individuals living with hemochromatosis.

These advancements may include:

1. **Genetic Research**: Ongoing genetic research may lead to a deeper understanding of the genetic factors that contribute to hemochromatosis. This knowledge could potentially pave the way for more

personalized treatment approaches.

2. **Treatment Innovations**: Advances in treatment options, such as new iron chelators or therapies targeting specific aspects of iron metabolism, may offer improved management options.

3. **Improved Diagnostics**: More accurate and accessible diagnostic tools could lead to earlier detection and intervention, reducing the risk of complications.

4. **Awareness and Advocacy**: Continued efforts to raise awareness about hemochromatosis can lead to increased funding for research, improved access to healthcare, and better support for individuals with the condition.

5. **Telemedicine and Remote Monitoring**: The integration of telemedicine and remote monitoring technologies may enhance the management of hemochromatosis, allowing for more convenient and

frequent check-ins with healthcare providers.

By emphasizing the importance of staying informed about the latest developments in hemochromatosis management, this chapter can empower individuals to take an active role in their health and stay hopeful about the future.

CONCLUSION

In closing, this book on hemochromatosis diet and management provides a comprehensive guide to understanding, addressing, and living well with this condition. From the basics of hemochromatosis and dietary guidelines to lifestyle strategies, emotional support, and the latest advances in research, this book aims to equip individuals with the knowledge and resources needed to effectively manage their health.

Living with hemochromatosis may present challenges, but with the right information, support, and a proactive approach to health, individuals can lead fulfilling lives while effectively managing their condition.